ALKALINE SMOOTHIES

A Beginner's Guide for Women on Managing
Weight Loss and Increasing Energy Through
Alkaline Smoothies, With Curated Recipes

Mary Golanna

mindplusfood

CONTENTS

DISCLAIMER

By reading this disclaimer, you are accepting the terms of the disclaimer in full. If you disagree with this disclaimer, please do not read the guide.

All of the content within this guide is provided for informational and educational purposes only, and should not be accepted as independent medical or other professional advice. The author is not a doctor, physician, nurse, mental health provider, or registered nutritionist/dietician. Therefore, using and reading this guide does not establish any form of a physician-patient relationship.

Always consult with a physician or another qualified health provider with any issues or questions you might have regarding any sort of medical condition. Do not ever disregard any qualified professional medical advice or delay seeking that advice because of anything you have read in this guide. The information in this guide is not intended to be any sort of medical advice and should not be used in lieu of any medical advice by a licensed and qualified medical professional.

The information in this guide has been compiled from a variety of known sources. However, the author cannot attest to or guarantee the accuracy of each source and thus should not be held liable for any errors or omissions.

You acknowledge that the publisher of this guide will not be held liable for any loss or damage of any kind incurred as a result of this guide or the reliance on any information provided within this guide. You acknowledge and agree that you assume all risk and responsibility for any action you undertake in response to the information in this guide.

Using this guide does not guarantee any particular result (e.g., weight loss or a cure). By reading this guide, you acknowledge that there are no guarantees to any specific outcome or results you can expect.

All product names, diet plans, or names used in this guide are for identification purposes only and are the property of their respective owners. The use of these names does not imply endorsement. All other trademarks cited herein are the property of their respective owners.

Where applicable, this guide is not intended to be a substitute for the original work of this diet plan and is, at most, a supplement to the original work for this diet plan and never a direct substitute. This guide is a personal expression of the facts of that diet plan.

Where applicable, persons shown in the cover images are stock photography models and the publisher has obtained the rights to use the images through license agreements with third-party stock image companies.

INTRODUCTION

Back in 2013, Victoria Beckham, also known as Posh from the 90s British girl group Spice Girls, popularized the alkaline diet by sharing on Twitter the cookbook "Honestly Healthy: Eat with Your Body in Mind, the Alkaline Way" by Chef Natasha Corrett and nutritionist Vicki Edgson.

Soon after, everyone followed suit and made the alkaline diet the new diet trend of the year.

People did not stop raving about it and started coining it as the "anti-aging diet" after discovering and experiencing its benefits for the skin.

Theories suggest that by following an alkaline diet you can increase collagen synthesis for skin elasticity, reduce inflammation in the form of acne and skin allergy, and strengthen the skin barrier of those with dry and fragile skin.

This uptrend was hyped up even more by testimonies revolving around effective weight loss and improvement from health conditions such as acid reflux, indigestion, autoimmune diseases (e.g. rheumatoid arthritis, DM Type 1, etc.), and cancer.

It might sound a bit new, but did you know that this diet has been around since the 1920s?

A New York physician named Dr. William Howard Hay created the

Hay Diet way back in the 1920s. He categorized foods into acidic, alkaline, and neutral—promoting the proper combination of foods to avoid stomach illnesses and secondary chronic diseases.

Fast forward to today, Dr. Hay's diet is appreciated more than ever. Because apparently, research has found some scientific explanations for the concept of the Hay or Alkaline Diet.

This diet suggests that by helping our body maintain our normal pH (~7.365), we can lessen the workload and stress on the body, eventually conserving more energy. In turn, the body can steer clear of chronic diseases, achieve normal body weight, and promote overall health.
If you want to reset your health and want a diet that will help you gain more energy, lose weight, or address a certain health condition, read further.

In this guide, you will...
• Learn what the alkaline diet is all about.
• Discover the health benefits of an alkaline diet in women.
• Determine how the alkaline diet can help you lose weight and gain more energy
• Familiarize yourself with alkaline ingredients.
• Learn how to begin incorporating alkaline smoothies into your diet

ALKALINE DIET 101

You probably have an idea what this diet is all about, but just can't put your finger on it. Sometimes called the alkaline ash diet or acid-alkaline diet, this diet is more of a holistic approach to health rather than a change in eating habits alone.

As the name implies, it promotes a more alkaline environment for the body, which involves switching acid-forming foods for alkaline-forming foods. Wherein, 70% is alkaline and 30% is acidic.

Usually, the confusion begins in differentiating acidic sources from alkaline sources. But do not worry because more of this will be tackled later on.

There may be some similarities to a vegan diet due to the preference for vegetables and fruits. Except that it is more specific to the pH of the food and provides a 30% leeway for meats and dairy.

What are some examples of alkaline-forming foods?

These are:
• Green leafy vegetables
• Coconut or almond milk
• Plant-based protein
• Almonds

• Seeds (e.g. chia and flax)

Whereas, the acidic-promoting foods to reduce are:
• Dairy
• Eggs
• Meat
• Processed food
• Refined sugar
• Caffeine
• Alcohol
• Some sources of carbohydrates such as grains, cereals, and oats

Carbohydrates may look alkaline, but they are acid-forming. The grains contain phytates that bind to phosphorus. And this binding prevents the blood from raising blood pH levels. Hence, making them acid-generating foods.

Aside from this, carbohydrates have the potential to block minerals from being absorbed properly when combined with other foods. Which gives us more reason to control our intake of carbohydrates.

The Alkaline Diet and the Acid-Ash Hypothesis
Now that you have an idea of what an alkaline diet is, let us dive deeper into what alkaline means.

Chemists and researchers use "pH" as a measurement to tell whether something is acidic or alkaline. It is a scale that ranges from 0 to 14 where 0 is the most acidic and 14 is the most alkaline (or basic).

It is considered alkaline if it falls within the range of 7.1–14.0. Whereas, acid refers to 0.0–6.9 pH.

What does this have to do with our human body?

Our bodies, as complex as they are, have different pH levels for every system. For example, our stomach is normal at low pH (acidic) to break down the food that we eat and to protect our gut from opportunistic microorganisms. Whereas, our blood is normal at an alkaline pH (7.36 to 7.44) that keeps the pH levels in our body balanced.

A jump outside the normal range can cause a ripple effect on other body parts, most especially the lungs and kidneys. And if the pH is left imbalanced for a long time, these areas can encounter serious complications.

So how does following an alkaline ash diet help?

The process of breaking down food is like setting something on fire—when it burns to make energy out of the food that you eat, some ash (our metabolic waste) is left behind.

Based on the acid-ash hypothesis, the pH of the ashcan alters the pH of the body. Meaning, if we eat acidic food and leave behind acidic ash, we can "acidify" our body's pH, which in theory can lead to diseases. And by following an alkaline diet, we can keep the pH of our body within normal levels.

However, this was clarified by Schwalfenberg et al. He and his team concluded from their study that eating acidic food does not directly affect the blood pH but the urine pH. And the health benefits observed from the alkaline diet stem from the fact that it is mostly composed of vegetables and fruits.

This is why the alkaline diet is considered more of a lifestyle rather than a strict diet. It will build the discipline for choosing the right kinds of foods.

HEALTH BENEFITS OF THE ALKALINE DIET

Alkaline for Women

Women are awesome in every way—they are the only ones who can menstruate, conceive, give birth to children, and juggle chores while staying pretty and presentable. They also have a special aptitude when it comes to nurturing relationships.

However, behind their strengths and capabilities, are physiological challenges that make their body more vulnerable to stress and other conditions compared to their male counterparts.

If you read further, you will discover how the alkaline diet can benefit women like you to have a healthier and more holistic lifestyle.

Beauty and Antiaging

As Corrett and Edgson mentioned in their book "Honestly Healthy for Life," eliminating acid-forming foods and toxins from the body can prevent general inflammation in the body. This alone can protect normal physiology and preserve the integrity of the skin.

How? When we eat too many refined sugars, the fructose and sucrose from these sugars bind to the amino acids in our skin collagen, and elastin through a process called glycation.

This binding of sugars to our skin's amino acids produces AGEs (Advanced Glycation End Products). What makes this a problem is that we cannot "unbind" them. This is why we can use them as biomarkers for aging.

So, the more sugars you consume, the higher your AGEs will be, and the faster you will age. Which results in a decrease in elasticity, slower wound healing, and uneven distribution of vessels in the dermis of the skin.

Since the alkaline diet abstains from refined sugars and is mostly composed of antioxidants, fatty acids, and other vitamins, following this diet can delay the formation of your AGEs. In turn, improving the clarity and suppleness of your skin. Hence, coining it as the "antiaging diet."

Reflux Disease
Reflux diseases are supposed to be as common in women as it is in men. But recently, there have been more cases of reflux disease in women.

One of the most obvious benefits of the alkaline diet is relief from Gastroesophageal Reflux (GERD) and Laryngopharyngeal Reflux (LPR).

In uncontrolled GERD and LPR, a digestive enzyme that is used to break down proteins in the gut, called pepsin, can cause damage to the esophagus and larynx.

This enzyme is stable at pH 7.4 and is activated by acid or Hydrogen ions.

Koufman et al. discovered that pH 8.8 alkaline water can permanently alter pepsin reducing potential damage in the esophagus and larynx suggesting that drinking alkaline water can be an additional treatment for patients who suffer from reflux disease.

Kidney Function
Did you know that according to the estimate of the Centers for Disease Control and Prevention (CDC) of the United States, Chronic Kidney Disease (CKD) is more common in women than in men?

The risk of acquiring a kidney disease in women increases during pregnancy, especially during the early stages.

There is a condition called pre-eclampsia; wherein, your blood pressure spikes up without prior notice during pregnancy. If left unmanaged, the increase in blood pressure can decrease the supply of blood to your organs causing irreversible damage, most especially to your liver and kidneys. This is why your obstetrician needs to monitor your blood pressure when you are pregnant.

Passey et al. discovered that an alkaline plant-based diet can reduce the workload on the kidneys of patients with Chronic Kidney Disease, eventually slowing down the progression of the disease.

This claim was supported by Yari and the company, saying that by consuming more vegetables and fruits, you can keep kidney biomarkers within normal levels and decrease acid residues or what we call "ash."

Some even say that a plant-based diet has the potential to improve the survival of patients with End-Stage Kidney Damage (ESKD).

Although more evidence is needed to prove the effectiveness of the alkaline diet on the kidneys, there is no harm in practicing preventive measures.

Breast Cancer
Breast cancer is the most prevalent cancer among American

women. The American Cancer Society claims that 1 out of 8 American women has a chance of developing breast cancer.

Some findings demonstrate the association between a high acid load in the diet and an increased risk of invasive breast cancer.

By lowering the acid load in your diet, you can control your risk of developing invasive breast cancer. Particularly, breast cancer patients who are estrogen receptor-negative—a kind of breast cancer where cells continue to grow even when medicated with hormone therapy drugs.

Other Cancers
Regardless of whether you have a family history of cancer, are a cancer patient, or just want to be healthier, it would be smart to take heed of the advice that a diet predominantly plant-based can decrease your risk of developing cancer.

The evidence-based medical guidelines recommend cancer patients keep a diet that is mostly plant-based while staying away from meat and processed foods which is very similar to the alkaline diet.

Muscle Mass Index
No matter how heavy women lift or how often they work out, without supplementation, women will not grow as much muscle as men.
The genetic makeup of men makes it easy for them to gain muscle mass much easier than women.

This becomes more challenging as women approach menopause. Muscle and bone loss become more evident as estrogen levels decline.

This is why aside from exercise and supplements, diet plays a big role in muscle mass and bone strength.

Meat provides an abundant source of protein. However, theories suggest that it contributes to the acidity of the body. Wherein, a good alternative would be protein-rich vegetables that can provide, not only protein but also potassium and magnesium. This provides proper nutrition to generate an adequate amount of energy for the body to function at its maximum potential.

One study shows that there is a positive correlation between an alkaline plant-based diet and muscle mass preservation in healthy women.

Overall Health
Based on the findings of Schwalfenberg, et. al., consumption of fruits and vegetables has positive effects on the following:
• Potassium-Sodium ratio in our body
• Bone health
• Muscle mass preservation
• Prevention of age-related diseases
• Growth hormone levels
• Cardiovascular health
• Memory
• Cognition

Alkaline for Weight Loss
Given the restrictions in the diet, you can expect to lose excess fat faster and more effectively. One such example is simply replacing your usual processed snacks with almonds.

This practice alone can lower your cholesterol levels and shed some weight. How? Salt from junk foods increases water retention in the body which adds up to your body weight.

They can also contain a lot of simple sugars that contribute to insulin spikes. These spikes are a response to sugar intake to make energy out of the sugar. However, frequent occurrences of insulin spikes can lead to diabetes and weight gain.

This is why most junk and fast food have empty calories—they contain a lot of calories but do not offer a lot of nutrition for the body.

Another example is avocados. Since it contains oleic acid, it can make you full fast and prevent you from munching on snacks. What makes this a better option is that it contains LDL which is a healthy fat that can lower your cholesterol levels.

Alkaline for Energy
Two theories explain the association between an alkaline diet and energy. The first theory claims that when the body is too acidic, it autopilots and goes through a protective mechanism.

Some individuals retain water. Whereas others do the opposite by flushing out water to protect their organs from too much acid. Either or, this defensive mechanism consumes a lot of energy that could be used for normal functioning.

The second theory suggests that the alteration in the pH of the gut makes it more susceptible for yeast and bacteria to thrive. This is supposed to be harmless except that these pathogens compete with the body for energy. This is why eating more does not always equate to gaining more energy.

STARTING THE ALKALINE DIET

C ontrary to popular belief, this diet is more than just a fad. You can reap the benefits or reach your health and weight loss goals if you can commit to following its restrictions.

A one-week routine will not provide maximum results. For you to experience the benefits, you need to give it time and patience. Before you begin, you need to promise yourself that you will stay for good. Unless of course your physician or nutritionist advises you otherwise.

If and when you slip, do not give up. Forgive yourself and continue trying. Always remind yourself of why you started in the first place—it may be for health purposes or a more holistic lifestyle. This will help you stay on course.

How do you begin then? Some can go cold turkey right away, while others like to dip their toes first. Going cold turkey will require dropping everything that is not on the list all at once. However, if you think that's too much for you, one way of going about it is by starting with "Meatless Mondays" where you start removing sources of meat every Monday and replacing it with a protein-rich salad.

Once you get the hang of this, you can gradually increase the frequency until you're able to do it daily. On top of this, you can start replacing your breakfast and usual snacks with an alkaline smoothie on your meatless days until you can do this daily.

In the next chapter, you will familiarize yourself with alkaline ingredients and learn how to prepare alkaline smoothies.

WEEK 1 OF THE ALKALINE DIET

Get-to-Know the Ingredients

The reason why a smoothie is a good start is that it is an easy way of consuming 4 to 5 servings of vegetables effortlessly daily.

Even if you are removing your meat, dairy, and some carbohydrates, you still need to be able to provide the same amount of nutrition for your body to function properly. This means that you need to keep up with the recommended daily allowance in the form of mostly vegetables and fruits. This is possible by eating more.

However, eating 5 to 6 meals a day or having big bowls thrice a day might not be feasible for everyone. So having a smoothie once or twice a day might do the trick. Plus, it's flavorful, handy, and can help familiarize your palate with the taste of vegetables and fruits.

As mentioned earlier, an alkaline smoothie contains fruits and vegetables. However, alkaline-forming foods are not easily distinguishable from acid-forming sources. You can always refer to an alkaline food chart for guidance. Here are some examples:

Highly alkaline fruits:

- lemon
- lime
- avocado
- grapefruit
- coconut
- tomato

Acidic fruits:
neutral to mildly acidic
- cantaloupe
- currants
- fresh dates
- nectarine
- plum
- sweet cherry
- watermelon

moderately acidic
- strawberry
- apple
- grapes
- apricot
- banana
- mango
- peach
- blackberry
- cranberry
- mangosteen
- apricot
- orange
- papaya
- blueberry
- pineapple

Green vegetables:
- kale

- spinach
- lettuce
- cabbage

Seeds:
- hemp
- flax
- chia

As you can see, citrus fruits are still included on this list. It might be a bit confusing because of their acidic pH and sour taste. But they promote an alkaline pH once broken down because of the potassium that they leave behind in your system.

Meaning, the fruit itself is acidic but is alkaline-forming inside the body. So even if they are categorized under "slightly or moderately acidic," you can still add them to your grocery list.

Plus, citrus fruits contain large amounts of antioxidants. So removing them from the diet would be such a waste.

If you're still worried about their acidity despite them being alkaline-promoting, adding non-dairy milk can help increase the pH of the smoothie. This is why most alkaline smoothie recipes suggest the addition of non-dairy milk especially when berries and citrus fruits are part of the recipe.

Also, do remember that the alkaline diet is not an all-or-nothing diet. You just need to stick to the 70/30 rule, where 70% is alkaline and the remaining 30% may or may not be acid. This is where you can insert your whole bread, wheat, oats, and brown rice.

Skip the Acids
Purge your cabinets of anything tempting. That may be any of the following:
- Carbonated beverages: soda, seltzer, or spritzers

- Alcohol
- Dairy milk
- Coffee and tea
- Sugar and sweeteners

Remember, it is easy to forget about them if they are out of sight.

Invest in a Blender

How can you make a smoothie without a blender?

If you don't have one yet, it's about time that you purchase one. You'll be needing this daily once you start adding alkaline smoothies to your diet every day.

Here are a few things to take note of while choosing which blender to get:

1. There are two kinds of blenders: countertop and hand blenders. For smoothies, opt for the countertop.

2. There are different kinds of containers: glass, plastic, and stainless steel. You can choose whichever tickles your fancy. Just make sure that it's BPA-free because it is a harmful chemical that can be absorbed by your food.

3. The most important feature to look at is the power of the motor. High-end blenders can easily crush ice cubes even at their slowest speed, while some budget-friendly ones require diluting them with water. This single feature will greatly influence the consistency of your smoothie.

4. Before adding it to your shopping cart, ask about its durability. The motor should be able to withstand daily use without requiring frequent repair.

Wirecutter's top picks would be Vitamix 5200, Oster Versa Pro Series Blender, Cleanblend Blender, and Oster Versa Pro Series Blender. Other good options would be Ninja Blender and

MARY GOLANNA

Nutribullet.

WEEK 2 OF THE ALKALINE DIET

Learn How to Prep
Plan the smoothies you want to have for next week so that you can make a list of what to buy from the grocery.

Here is a sample schedule that you can follow while getting the hang of it:

DAY	SMOOTHIE
MONDAY	Fruity Berry Spinach
TUESDAY	Kale Mango Smoothie
WEDNESDAY	Spinach Berry Lemon Smoothie
THURSDAY	Grapefruit and Spinach Smoothie
FRIDAY	Veggie Blast Smoothie
SATURDAY	Pomegranate Refreshing Smoothie

Once you have all the ingredients you'll need, you can move on to prepping.

Although experts usually do this on Sundays, you can designate any day of the week for preparing the ingredients of your smoothies. Besides, it will only take 1 to 2 hours of your time.

Step 1: Pack the ingredients in reusable plastic or Tupperware. Just make sure that if you prefer a Ziploc, choose the freezer bag because the material is thicker and can preserve the ingredients longer.

Step 2: If it's in plastic, squeeze out the air and seal properly.

Step 3: Label them accordingly—it may be the corresponding day of the week or the name of the smoothie.

Step 4: Freeze at least a night before consumption to produce smoother consistency.

This way, on the day itself, you can just dump everything into the blender and save time.

WEEK 3 OF THE ALKALINE DIET

Before diving in, here are just some tips to consider when making your shake:

Frozen fruit is better than ice.
As mentioned earlier, this will give your shake a thicker consistency and a more even taste compared to just dumping it with ice.

Add more liquid.
If it's too thick, don't be scared to add liquid gradually. You can do this by adding one scoop at a time.

Low-High-Low.
Start blending at a low speed. Then, slowly increase. Once you're about to reach your preferred consistency, gradually switch back to a slower speed.

Instagram-worthy color.
If you want to prevent your shake from turning brown and instead want it to be visually catchy, say for Instagram, remember not to blend the red/purple concoction with the greens. It's a bit of a stretch but you have to blend them separately. Only mix them once ready to drink.

Once ready, you can now start blending your shake. You can take this either for breakfast or an afternoon snack. And since it's heavy on fiber, you can expect the shake to keep you full for at least two hours.

Below are the recipes for the smoothies mentioned in the previous chapter.

Enjoy!

SAMPLE RECIPES

Fruity Berry Spinach Smoothie

Ingredients:
- 1 cup watermelon
- 1 cup almond milk
- 1/2 small banana
- 1 handful of spinach
- 5 frozen strawberries
- 1 tsp. chia seeds
- 1 cup ice

Instructions:
1. Mix spinach, banana, chia seeds, half cup of ice, and a half cup of almond milk. Do this to prevent a brown smoothie.
2. Pour into a glass.
3. Blend the rest of the ingredients.
4. Pour both of the mixtures into the same glass.
5. Serve and enjoy!

Kale Mango Smoothie

Ingredients:
- 2 large kale leaves, washed
- 1 banana
- 1 handful of spinach, washed
- 1/2 cup mango, frozen and chopped
- 1 lemon
- 2 pcs. thumb-sized ginger knobs
- 1 cup water

Instructions:
1. Peel the lemon.
2. Toss all ingredients into the blender. Blend for about a minute, until smooth.
3. Serve and enjoy.

Spinach Berry Lemon Smoothie

Ingredients:
- 2 cups fresh spinach leaves, rinsed and roughly chopped
- 7–8 frozen strawberries
- 1 tbsp. chia seeds
- 1 tbsp. lemon juice
- 1 frozen banana, sliced
- 2–3 cups coconut water, chilled

Instructions:
1. Put the spinach leaves into the blender.
2. Add the banana, strawberries, lemon juice, chia seeds, and coconut water.
3. Blend well.
4. Serve and enjoy!

Grapefruit and Spinach Smoothie

Ingredients:
- 1 grapefruit
- 1 cup coconut milk
- 1 cup spinach
- a pinch of Stevia to sweeten

Instructions:
1. Put all the ingredients in the blender.
2. Blend well.
3. Serve and enjoy.

Veggie Blast Smoothie

Ingredients:
- 4 tomatoes
- 1 cucumber
- 1 garlic clove
- 1/2 cup rosemary infusion
- 1/2 onion
- 1 tbsp. virgin olive oil
- 1 lemon juice
- 1 cup of spinach or kale juice
- Himalayan salt, to taste
- black pepper, to taste

Instructions:
1. Blend and mix with spinach juice and lemon juice.
2. Add salt and pepper to taste.
3. Serve and enjoy.

Pomegranate Refreshing Smoothie

Ingredients:
- 2 grapefruits
- 1/2 pomegranate
- 3 large collard leaves
- 1 cup coconut water

Instructions:
1. Put all ingredients in a blender.
2. Blend well.
3. Serve and enjoy.

CONCLUSION

Thank you again for getting this guide.

If you found this guide helpful, please take the time to share your thoughts and post a review. It'd be greatly appreciated!

Thank you and good luck!

REFERENCES AND HELPFUL LINKS

5 most important things to consider before buying a blender. (n.d.). Retrieved December 24, 2022, from https://www.reviewsworthy.net/blenders/important-things-consider-buying-blender.

Amount of muscle mass in men versus women. (n.d.). LIVESTRONG.COM. Retrieved December 24, 2022, from https://www.livestrong.com/article/246036-how-much-more-muscle-mass-does-a-male-have-than-a-female/.

Breast cancer statistics | How common is breast cancer? (n.d.). Retrieved December 24, 2022, from https://www.cancer.org/cancer/breast-cancer/about/how-common-is-breast-cancer.html.

Clegg, D. J., & Hill Gallant, K. M. (2019). Plant-based diets in CKD. Clinical Journal of the American Society of Nephrology: CJASN, 14(1), 141–143. https://doi.org/10.2215/CJN.08960718.

Does food combining work? the hay diet - infofit - personal trainer certification. Infofit. (2022, September 22). Retrieved December 24, 2022, from https://infofit.ca/food-combining-work-hay-diet/.

Fast food's effects on 8 areas of the body. (2022, November 14). Healthline. https://www.healthline.com/health/fast-food-effects-on-body.

Healthfully. (n.d.). Healthfully. Retrieved December 24, 2022, from https://healthfully.com/300334-acid-forming-foods-vs-alkaline-forming-foods.html.

Koufman, J. A., & Johnston, N. (2012). Potential benefits of ph 8. 8 alkaline drinking water as an adjunct in the treatment of reflux disease. Annals of Otology, Rhinology & Laryngology, 121(7), 431–434. https://doi.org/10.1177/000348941212100702.

Nguyen, H. P., & Katta, R. (2015). Sugar sag: Glycation and the role of diet in aging skin. Skin Therapy Letter, 20(6), 1–5.

Nutrition. (n.d.). Byrdie. Retrieved December 24, 2022, from https://www.byrdie.com/nutrition-4628394.

Passey, C. (2017). Reducing the dietary acid load: How a more alkaline diet benefits patients with chronic kidney disease. Journal of Renal Nutrition: The Official Journal of the Council on Renal Nutrition of the National Kidney Foundation, 27(3), 151–160. https://doi.org/10.1053/j.jrn.2016.11.006

Schwalfenberg, G. K. (2012). The alkaline diet: Is there evidence that an alkaline ph diet benefits health? Journal of Environmental and Public Health, 2012, 1–7. https://doi.org/10.1155/2012/727630

Singh, S. (2021, April 15). Gastroesophageal reflux disease (Gerd) in women—Harvard. Steamdaily. https://steamdaily.com/gastroesophageal-reflux-disease-gerd-in-women-harvard/.

Sipilä, S., Törmäkangas, T., Sillanpää, E., Aukee, P., Kujala, U. M., Kovanen, V., & Laakkonen, E. K. (2020). Muscle and bone mass in middle-aged women: Role of menopausal status and physical activity. Journal of Cachexia, Sarcopenia and Muscle, 11(3), 698–709. https://doi.org/10.1002/jcsm.12547.

Yari, Z., & Mirmiran, P. (2018). Alkaline diet: A novel nutritional strategy in chronic kidney disease? Iranian Journal of Kidney Diseases, 12(4), 204–208.

Made in the USA
Las Vegas, NV
09 December 2024

13571695R00022